KETOGENIC DIET

35 Recipes for Rapid Weight Loss With This Amazing Low Carb, High Fat Diet (Ketogenic Diet Cookbook, Ketogenic Diet Recipes, Anti Inflammatory Diet)

By PAUL GUT

Table of Contents

Copyright Notice

Disclaimer

Introduction

Dietetics have been trying to convince us for decades that diet with little fat and a lot of starch (the food pyramid) will help us lose all fatty tissue from our body, but over 60% of the population in the United States still suffers from obesity. On the other side, there are growing evidence that reducing carbohydrate intake is the right way if you want to lose weight quickly and efficiently, without any negative consequences, and what is most important, with preserving the muscle mass. Therefore, Ketogenic diet definitely falls to ones of the most popular weight loss methods, which are now widely applied across the planet. The term "Ketogenic diet" includes meals that minimize carbohydrate intake during the day. This carb restriction leads our organism into a state of so-called ketosis, and then fatty tissue rapidly starts to disappear from your belly.

In following chapters I will explain everything you need to know about this diet and the easiest way how to successfully adhere to this diet regime. This diet is nowadays, most commonly used by bodybuilders (when they need to remove all excess fat "in a hurry"), so if you, for example, have some important social event in just two weeks by keeping this diet you will literally be halved. So, let's start.

What is Ketogenic diet?

Most of us, have probably heard by now that Ketogenic diet was developed to help people who suffer from epilepsy at first. Even a movie "Lorenzo's oil" was filmed with first steps of developing this kind of diet and Nick Nolte was one of the main actors. The first person, who named this kind of dieting as "Ketogenic diet" was Russel Wilder from the Mayo Clinic in 1921. Therefore, this diet isn't so "new" but in the last decade, it was wildly pronounced as diet against obesity. When our body is "forced" to use fats as the main source of energy ketones (kind of acids) start to produce in our body, because of the lack of carbs as a source of energy for proper work of our body . I must warn you that people who suffer from type 1 diabetes shouldn't apply this kind of dieting, because high levels of ketones can lead to the pathological ketoacidosis, but for everybody else, this kind of dieting is safe and the only thing what will occur is physiological ketosis and our body in such cases keeps production ketones under control.

Beneficial function of Ketogenic diet

Faster weight loss

You will lose weight much faster with Ketogenic diet than with any other kind of fasting and what is more important you will not be hungry at any moment with this kind of dieting. The main reason for this feeling of fluffiness is the ratio between fats, protein and carbs (4:1). This means that you can include any kind of healthy fats like butter, lard, olive oil or duck fat in your meals, and restrictions are linked with high carbo food like grains, pasta, bread, sugar, and fruits.

Forget type 2 diabetes

Insulin resistance is the main cause of getting type 2 diabetes with our habitual modern eating habits and with the Ketogenic diet you will avoid this condition. Insulin resistance appears when cells all over the body no longer respond to the insulin (hormone). This means that our organs, including muscles, have trouble absorbing glucose (the main source of energy) from blood and so sugar stays in our blood and pancreas continues producing more insulin. With Ketogenic diet intake of carbs is restricted therefore apparency of high sugar level in the bloodstream is disabled.

It stops development of many cardiovascular diseases

When it comes to the long-term Ketogenic dieting (at least 24 weeks), high level of bad cholesterol and triglyceride will significantly decrease. This means that you will prevent any development of atherosclerosis, and your blood vessels will not harden or tighten, so the risk of <u>heart attack</u> and <u>stroke</u> will be lowered as well.

It contributes against cancer

The essential ingredient for developing cancer cells in our body is sugar, so once again by lowering carb intake you will lower the chances of developing any kind of cancer. In the past few years, Ketogenic diet has even been included in cancer therapy because of its effect on decreasing of existed tumor mass.

At last but not least this diet has been used for over 100 years as a tool in the treatment of epilepsy seizures.

Chapter 1: The easiest way to adapt to Ketogenic diet

Whenever we try to change any of our acquired habits, we need to include a lot of effort to achieve it. Therefore, I will not tell you that it's easy to switch to Ketogenic diet, especially if you tried various kinds of diets that exclude a higher intake of fats for a longer period of time, and most diets nowadays are based on lower intake of fats. Almost nothing is unreachable and every habit is changeable. A little persistence, a bit of stubbornness and much of good will and you will very soon accept this new way of dieting.

If you like to eat meat than this change in your eating pattern will go much faster because you need to include all kinds of meat, fish, and seafood; fatty fish is a good choice for keeping a Ketogenic diet. Include red and white meat like beef, pork poultry, lamb, but you should avoid breaded meat and meat products like sausages, hot dogs or any kind of meat products that contain starch, sugar or sauces. You can even involve animal organs like liver, heart or kidneys, but only from grass fed animals. Meat presents a good source of proteins and healthy fats.

Eggs and fatty fish like salmon, tuna, sardines, mackerel, and trout should also be on your menu and from healthy fats real butter, lard, tallow, olive oil, coconut oil and seeds product in a form of butter, like peanut butter and tahini paste should be on your table every day, because they are very rich in omega 3 fatty acids.

From veggies, you should include non-starchy veggies like spinach, Swiss chard, lettuce, chard, endive, celery stalk, kohlrabi, zucchini, cucumber, asparagus and all other dark green veggies.

Fruits like all kinds of berries (strawberries, blackberries, blueberries, chokeberry raspberries) avocado, nuts, and seeds belong to low carbs food so they present the best choice when Ketogenic diet is in the matter. From other kinds of fruits, you can include watermelon, grapefruit, cantaloupe melon, raw apricot and Honeydew melon in moderate amounts.

You can begin this diet by avoiding bread and cereal products in the first week and in the second week exclude them completely. This will be one of the easiest ways to start with Ketogenic diet.

What food should you avoid

The main goal of the Ketogenic diet is to avoid food that is rich in carbohydrates (high in starch content and low in dietary fibers). This means that you should avoid all kinds of takeaway food, meat products, and products made from grains like wheat rye, barley, quinoa, oats, and bulgur in any form including pasta, pizza, cookies, sprouted grains and rice. From veggies, potatoes should also be excluded from your menu. Some fruits are also forbidden such as banana, pineapple, mango, grapes and from citrus fruit also avoid tangerine as much as you can because they also contain a higher amount of carbohydrate.

From beverages any kind of sugary soft drinks, energy drinks, beer and cocktails are limited in this kind of dieting. Intake of milk should be reduced to a minimum as it contains a higher amount of carbs, but you can involve it once or twice a week in moderate amounts (half a cup max), and don't worry about calcium intake while you can eat dairy products on a daily base.

Sweets in a form of processed food as ready–to-eat cakes, ice cream, puddings should stay on the shelf in the store but not in your home. So, even if some cravings appear you won't have it on your hand to eat it, and I really hope that you will be lazy to go to the store just for some candy.

Any kind of GMO products including soy and products that contain gluten (a protein that is a part of a wheat component) are forbidden in this diet, which is good because more and more people suffer from gluten sensitivity. Symptoms of gluten sensitivity include irritable bowel syndrome, bloating, stomach pain, diarrhea, tiredness, and in some cases it even causes depression.

First signs that your body has switched to ketosis condition.

The hardest part is the first few days until the body gets used to the lack of carbohydrates. Keep in mind that with only one meal rich in carbohydrates you will probably get out of ketosis condition and for returning into ketosis you will again probably need 2 days. Therefore, rather prefer to specify a shorter period of time like few weeks in which you will not violate this diet.

During the first week of holding these dietary measures some of following symptoms may appear such as fatigue, exhaustion, tiredness, sleepiness during the day. Even your breath could start to smell like acetone, do not worry it's just a phase that will pass. Specifically, it is a natural and completely harmless condition. The implementation of Ketogenic diet, over time leads to a decrease in appetite so weight loss starts without losing muscle mass.

How much carbs can is allowed to intake during Ketogenic diet

I need to emphases that the maximum intake of carbs during Ketogenic diet differs from person to person. Someone will switch into ketosis with intake of 100g of carbs during a day and someone will achieve it only if intake of carbs reduces to 20g per day. Usually, people who are more energetic and physically active can get into ketosis state even if they intake 100g of carbs during a day because they probably have more muscle mass than sedentary kind of people. My advice is that you start your reduced intake of carbs with consuming maximum of 50g per day. Stick to it for a week or two and then try to add a bit more carbs until you reach 100g per day.

As I previously mentioned, the simplest way is to eliminate intake of bread, pastries and sweets. After that, whenever you go to a store for food supplies, look more carefully on the labels of some specific products that you want to buy and seek how much of carbs that product contains. My advice is that you only buy raw food (meat, veggies), which you will prepare at home. Remember that almost all half-finished products or ready–to-eat meals, that you only need to heat in microwave contain a high amount of sugar, because one of the main roles of added sugar is to preserve and extend the shelf life of a finished product. Whenever you see a word on a label that at the end has – "ose " like glucose, sucrose, lactose, fructose, corn syrup and so on it means that this specific product contains added amounts of sugar.

Do not worry! You still have a big choice of food to intake even if your goal is 50g carbs per day.

Even so that term of so-called "net carb" isn't yet recognized as a legal definition by FDA, they represent the total carbohydrate content of the food minus the fiber content – it means sugar content of all carbohydrates value in some product, and that is what you need to count in this diet, because dietary fibers belong to the so-called "good" carbohydrates that our body can't digest, but they influence on the normalization and regulation of digestion.

You can intake even 45 cups of raw spinach or 7 cups of cooked as a side dish and even then you won't exceed the overall intake of 50g carbs per day. I really believe that none of us will enter more than one or two cups of veggies during a meal.

I choose some healthy kind of dairy products like Greek yogurt, cream cheese feta, cottage and Gouda which you can eat, you can drink milk in moderate amount but as you can see if you want to stay in ketosis then you definitely need to expel ice cream from your diet during this period.

Chapter 2: Ketogenic Diet for Weight Loss

If you want to comply this diet with the main goal of losing weight then you need to incorporate the right ratio between fats, proteins, and carbs in your diet. This is completely opposite from any other kind of restricted diet that you have ever applied. It means that you need to add some fats in every meal because the ratio of the intake of fat, protein and carbohydrates should be up to 75% of fats, 20% of proteins and 5% of net carbs. Additional fat in your food will sooner lead to a condition of satiety. It means if you, for example, for breakfast prepare scrambled eggs then you need to add a teaspoon of butter for each egg, or when you prepare salad you should add at least 4 tablespoons of olive oil in it. Every time you roast your steak it should marinate for at least 2 hours in oil or spread with a tablespoon of lard, for example. Also, you need to choose fatty kinds of meat like pork and fatty fish.

Choose organic food, and don't forget to add fats in the form of butter, coconut oil, lard in your diet. As in any other kind of proper nutrition, meals should be divided into 5 meals during a day, and because the higher amount of fats, don't forget to drink plenty of water. Also, it would be good if you could avoid alcohol and artificial sweetener because the point of this diet is to enter as much as you can real food, not the one that comes from the laboratory. Don't forget that a healthy lifestyle includes enough time for sleep (at least 7 hours), and some physical recreation.

What is the main differ between Ketogenic diet and other verses of low carbs diets

Whenever you hear the term "low carb diet" it means that you need to lower your intake of carbohydrates from 60% under 20%, but you don't need to lower it to 5% as Ketogenic diet requires. This means that most low carbs diet don't include that your body needs to go ketosis status and use ketones bodies as a source of energy i.e. to obtain the body to use fatty acids as its primary fuel source, not carbohydrates. In others, low carbs diet your body will still use glucose as the main source of energy. You don't count calories intake in the Ketogenic diet, the only thing that you count is an intake of carbohydrates. The lack of hunger is the most important difference between Ketogenic diet and all others low carbs diets. So, if you really want to apply Ketogenic diet then use just recipes for Ketogenic diet not the ones for low carb intake.

Any kind of fats contains a high amount of calories, so if you count calories in this diet you will probably pass out from the total calorie intake during the day, because don't forget that you need to include minimum 2 tbsp. of fat in every meal that you prepare.

From fats expel any trans fats (hydrogenated oils), in your diet such as margarine, packaged cookies, cakes, crackers, and coffee creamers, fried and battered food, because such fats will increase bad cholesterol level (LDL), and even create inflammatory process inner your body, which then can lead to higher risk of getting a stroke.

Chapter 3: Example of one day meal plan for Ketogenic diet

I engaged a nutritionist to provide a daily meal plan so you can see exactly how your meal plan should look like. Through this pattern, you can very easily bring your body into a ketoses state. No bread, grains, and purchasable snacks. You won't make any mistakes if you add 2 to 4 tablespoons of oil in every salad that is mostly made from green veggies. For breakfast, you can choose canned fish, scrambled eggs with various kinds of veggies, roasted bacon or cheese, use your imagination, look over the net and I am sure that you will find many great recipes there.

Breakfast: Scrambled eggs with mushrooms

Preparation Time – 5 minutes
Cooking Time – 4 minutes
Serves – 1

<u>Ingredients:</u>

- 2 Large Eggs
- 2 Tablespoon of unsalted butter
- pinch of salt

- 2 oz of sliced mushrooms

Preparation:

1. Use a fork to beat the eggs together.
2. Melt the butter in medium nonstick skillet oven on low heat. Add sliced mushrooms and cook for a couple of minutes, until the liquid evaporates.
3. Add egg mixture.
4. Cook, continually moving eggs with the spatula, just until eggs are set, 2 to 3 minutes.
5. Season with salt; serve hot.

Nutritional facts: This meal contains 359 calories, 33.1g of fats, 14.6g of proteins, 1.8g of carbs from whom 0.6g are dietary fibers.

Snack I: a cup of raspberries

Nutritional facts: 64 calories, 0.8g fats, 1.5g proteins, 14.7g carbs from whom 8.0g are dietary fibers.

Lunch: Chicken breast in sauce of avocado

Preparation Time – 10 minutes
Cooking Time – 25 minutes
Serves -1
Ingredients:

- 1tbsp. of chopped onion

- 2 tbsp. of sliced mushrooms
- 1 large avocado
- 3 tablespoons lemon juice
- 2 tbsp. of sour cream
- 4 oz of chicken breast
- 3 tablespoons of olive oil
- 2 tablespoons of butter

Preparation:

1. First, make the sauce: fry chopped onion on a medium heated stove with 2 tbsp of olive oil, add the mushrooms and fry everything for a few minutes.
2. Cut avocado into cubes and pour lemon juice over so it doesn't go dark.
3. Then add the avocado with lemon juice in the saucepan and cook for a few minutes.
4. Remove from heat and finally, add sour cream. Set aside.
5. Heat 1 tbsp of oil with 2 tbsp of butter in another pan, when butter is melted add meat and cook for about 10 minutes. Remove from the stove, pour the sauce and serve.

Nutritional facts: This meal contains 1228 calories, 113.7g of fats, 42.0g of proteins, 20.5g of carbs from whom 14.0g are dietary   fibers.

Snack II: Homemade Cheesecake

Preparation Time – 5 minutes
Cooking Time – a minute
Serves -8

Ingredients:

- 38 oz of cream cheese
- ½ a cup of Stevia Sweetener
- 1 teaspoons of vanilla
- 2 tbsp of sour cream
- 4 eggs

Preparation:

1. Preheat the oven to 350°F/180°C.

2. Beat cream cheese in a bowl until fluffy, it takes a couple of minutes. Stir in liquid form of Stevia sweetener, mix a bit more and then add sour cream and vanilla extract, mixing all the time for a few more minutes.

3. Add eggs one by one mixing all the time. Beat until the fill thickness and becomes creamy, it will take approximately 5 minutes for all eggs to combine into the mixture.

4. Lightly grease the pan (9 spring form pan) and pour in the prepared mass. Put the springform on a baking sheet and bake

for 20 minutes or until puffy and lightly brown around the edges.

5. Let it cool before you put it in a fridge. Cover and chill for at least 4 hours.

Nutritional facts: This cake contains 509 calories, 49.8g of fats, 13.0g of proteins, and 3.9g of carbs per serving.

Dinner: Mixed Tuna Salad

Preparation Time – 15 minutes
Cooking Time – 8 minutes
Serves – 1

Ingredients:

- 1 Cup of chopped Lettuce
- 2 Hard Boiled Sliced Eggs
- 1 oz of Feta Cheese
- 2 oz of Shredded Cheese
- 1 medium sized Chopped Tomato
- 2 tbsp of Chopped Onions
- 1/2 of a Small Sliced Avocado
- 1 can of Tuna in oil
- 2 tbsp of Real Mayonnaise
- 1 tbsp of sour cream
- Pinch of Salt and Pepper

Preparation:

1. Pour cold water into a saucepan and put eggs, turn on the stove on high temperature and when it starts to boil, cook for another 5 minutes.

2. Cool, peel, slice them and mix with all ingredients except Mayonnaise and Sour Cream.

3. Separately stir these 2 ingredients, until they unit, add salt and pepper and pour over the salad.

Nutritional facts: This meal contains 1144 calories, 80.3g of fats, 80.8g of proteins, 27.5g of carbs from whom 9.0g are dietary fibers.

For the whole day you will enter: 3304 calories, 277.7g of fats, 151.9g of proteins, 68.4 of carbohydrates from whom 31.6g belong to dietary fibers which means that you will enter only 36.8g of net carbs. **This means that you have entered 75% of fats, 18.3% of proteins and 7% of totally carbohydrates intake or 1.04% of net carbs.** The ideal ratio in the Ketogenic diet of fat, protein and carbohydrates intake should be: 75% of fats, 20% of proteins and 5% of net carbs. So, through this example, I have shown you that you can even intake a dessert as a snack and if you follow this pattern of a meal plan you will achieve the ideal ratio of fats as average intake during a week.

I think that it would be much better if you prepare your own mayonnaise if you like such kind of food, because only then you can be sure that the artificial ingredients or hidden sugars aren't a part of this kind of grocery. It will really not take a lot of your free time for this and it will provide you a greater opportunity to combine ingredients and diverse menu as real mayonnaise can be added to any kind of salad or sauce. You can make mayo from any kind of seeds oil you prefer, I have chosen the olive oil because it belongs to healthier kinds of oil while it contains monounsaturated fatty acids known as "MUFAs". This specific kind of fatty acid acts directly on lowering the bad cholesterol level in your bloodstream and it also regulates your blood sugar level so that's why olive oil is always recommended to people who suffer from diabetes type2 and most importantly olive oil may increase longevity and reduce any aging process.

Homemade mayonnaise
Preparation Time – 15 minutes
Cooking Time –0 minutes
 Serves – 10

Ingredients:

- 4 large organic egg yolk
- 1 freshly squeezed lemon juice
- 1 tbsp. of white wine vinegar

- ½ a tsp of Dijon mustard
- ½ a tsp of salt
- ½ a cup olive oil

Preparation:

1. All ingredients for preparing a homemade mayo need to be at room temperature. This is really important for the emulsification process.

2. Put separated eggs yolks in a mixing bowl and mix it thoroughly, add lemon juice, vinegar, mustard, and salt, stirring constantly. Whisk until blended and bright yellow, about 2 more minutes.

3. First stir in slowly a few drops of oil, mixing constantly and then gradually pour in the rest of the oil whisking constantly until the mayo becomes thick. It will take about 10 more minutes. Keep in a fridge until serving.

Note: Mayonnaise will clot if you add the oil too quickly at the beginning. Also, *to avoid the risk of salmonella infection use only fresh organic eggs.*

Conclusion

This kind of dieting is an excellent choice for anybody who wants to lose extra fat and still preserve muscle mass in a short time. What's more important with this dieting you will not be hungry at any moment and you will even achieve a better blood picture in every aspect. This means that even though you will enter more fats, you will lower your bad cholesterol and triglyceride levels.

This kind of diet is an excellent choice, not just for people who suffers from extra weight, but for anyone who want to stay in better physical condition regardless of age. Only two weeks in every couple of months of this kind of dieting will help you avoid many serious diseases.

The Ketogenic diet is one the best ways of detoxification the body from many added artificial nutrients that we enter on a daily base in higher amounts, so if you want to help your heart, kidneys, liver, brain and overall bloodstream include this kind of dieting at least 3 times per year. I am sure that anyone can follow this kind of eating for 2 weeks. Don't eat just meat, fish, and eggs, you need to include food rich in dietary fibers content that can be found in many veggies and berries in your everyday meal plan because they are also full of important vitamins and antioxidants.

Never keep out of your mind that lack of fiber in nutrition leads to many uncomfortable physical conditions such as constipation or laziness of intestine, which then will endanger detoxification process in your body. So, try to include next ingredients in every meal: broccoli, green beans, cucumber, zucchini, lettuce salad, spinach, mushrooms, Swiss chard, because these veggies are included in every Ketogenic diet. It doesn't matter if you will involve them as a side dish or as a part of the main meal, always pour a serving or two of healthy fats over it, to ensure the ketosis condition.

www.ingramcontent.com/pod-product-compliance
Lightning Source LLC
Chambersburg PA
CBHW061949280526
45787CB00004B/1788